Colitis Diet Guide for Beginners

Importance of Diet in Managing Colitis

By

Cian Darroch

Table of Contents

CHAPTER 1

Introduction to Colitis Diet

1.1 Overview of Colitis

Colitis, broadly defined as inflammation of the colon, encompasses various conditions affecting the large intestine's lining. One of the primary types of colitis is Ulcerative Colitis (UC), an inflammatory bowel disease characterized by chronic inflammation and ulcers in the colon and rectum. Another form is Crohn's disease, which involves inflammation that extends through the entire digestive tract, often affecting different parts of the gastrointestinal system.

Nature of Colitis: Colitis presents a range of symptoms, including abdominal pain, diarrhea, rectal bleeding, weight loss, fatigue, and, in severe cases, complications like bowel perforation or strictures. These symptoms significantly impact the individual's quality of life, leading to discomfort and disruptions in daily activities.

Challenges Faced by Patients: Patients grappling with colitis often confront challenges in managing their condition, including unpredictable flare-ups, medication side effects, and the need for frequent medical evaluations. The symptoms' variability can create a profound impact on mental health, contributing to anxiety, depression, and social isolation.

Role of Diet in Colitis Management: Understanding the interplay between diet and colitis is crucial. While diet alone doesn't cause colitis, it can influence the frequency and severity of flare-ups. Certain foods might exacerbate symptoms, while others can aid in managing inflammation and supporting overall gut health. Consequently, adopting an appropriate diet tailored to an individual's needs becomes pivotal in managing and alleviating colitis symptoms.

Individualized Approach to Diet: It's essential to note that there's no one-size-fits-all diet for colitis. What works for one person may not be suitable for another due to the condition's variability and individual sensitivities. Therefore, developing a personalized dietary plan, often in collaboration with healthcare providers, dietitians, or gastroenterologists, is crucial to optimizing symptom management and improving overall well-being.

Holistic Management Approach: Beyond diet, managing colitis often involves a multi-faceted approach. Medications, lifestyle modifications, stress management, regular medical check-ups, and understanding triggers play pivotal roles in comprehensive colitis management. The diet acts as a fundamental component, working synergistically with other strategies to minimize symptoms and enhance the patient's quality of life.

comprehending colitis involves recognizing its diverse manifestations, acknowledging the impact on an individual's life, and appreciating the potential influence of diet in managing symptoms. An informed, tailored approach to diet forms an integral part of holistic colitis management, aiming to mitigate symptoms and improve the patient's overall health and well-being.

1.2 Importance of Diet in Managing Colitis

Diet plays a pivotal role in managing colitis due to its direct influence on gastrointestinal health and inflammation. Understanding the importance of diet in colitis management involves acknowledging its impact on symptom severity, flare-ups, and overall well-being.

Influence on Symptoms: Certain foods can trigger or exacerbate colitis symptoms. These triggers vary among individuals, but commonly reported culprits include high-fiber foods, spicy dishes, dairy products, caffeine, alcohol, and high-fat items. Additionally, some individuals might find relief by avoiding specific food groups or following diets that reduce inflammation in the gut.

Impact on Inflammation: Chronic inflammation characterizes colitis, and dietary choices can either contribute to or alleviate this inflammation. Foods rich in antioxidants, omega-3 fatty acids, and certain vitamins and minerals exhibit anti-inflammatory properties, potentially aiding in reducing gut inflammation. Conversely, processed foods, refined sugars, and trans fats may promote inflammation, worsening colitis symptoms.

Gut Microbiota and Diet: The gut microbiota, a community of beneficial bacteria in the digestive tract, plays a crucial role in gut health. Diet profoundly influences this microbiota composition. A colitis-friendly diet often focuses on promoting a balanced and diverse gut microbiome, which is associated with reduced inflammation and better overall gut health.

Individualized Dietary Approaches: Due to the unique nature of colitis triggers and tolerances, there's no universal diet regimen that suits everyone. Patients often benefit from keeping detailed food journals to identify personal triggers and patterns, allowing them to tailor their diets to manage symptoms effectively. This personalized approach enables individuals to find a dietary plan that suits their specific needs, minimizing discomfort and flare-ups.

1.3 Goals of a Colitis Diet Plan

A colitis diet plan aims to achieve several key objectives, focusing on improving symptoms, reducing inflammation, and supporting overall health:

Symptom Management: The primary goal of a colitis diet plan is to manage and alleviate symptoms such as abdominal pain, diarrhea, bloating, and rectal bleeding. Identifying trigger foods and eliminating or reducing their intake forms a fundamental aspect of symptom management.

Reducing Inflammation: By incorporating anti-inflammatory foods and avoiding those that promote inflammation, a colitis diet plan aims to minimize gut inflammation. This can potentially reduce the frequency and severity of flare-ups and contribute to long-term disease management.

Nutritional Support: Ensuring adequate nutrition is vital for individuals with colitis, as malabsorption, nutrient deficiencies, and weight loss are common concerns. A well-designed colitis diet plan focuses on providing essential nutrients, vitamins, and minerals while taking into account dietary restrictions or sensitivities.

Gut Health Optimization: Promoting a healthy gut microbiome through diet is a key aspect of colitis management. The diet plan may include foods that support beneficial gut bacteria, such as probiotics, prebiotics, and fiber-rich foods, fostering a balanced and thriving gut environment.

Individualized Approach: Recognizing the unique nature of colitis in each individual, the diet plan should be highly personalized. It adapts to an individual's triggers, preferences, and tolerances, empowering them to manage their condition effectively while maintaining a satisfying and sustainable diet.

a well-crafted colitis diet plan aims to alleviate symptoms, reduce inflammation, support optimal nutrition, and cater to the individual needs of those managing this chronic condition. Collaboration with healthcare professionals and a mindful, individualized approach to dietary changes are crucial elements in achieving these goals.

CHAPTER 2

Understanding Colitis

2.1 Types of Colitis: Ulcerative Colitis vs. Crohn's Disease

Ulcerative Colitis:

- **Location of Inflammation:** Primarily affects the colon and rectum.

- **Nature of Inflammation:** Continuous inflammation starts from the rectum and spreads upward into the colon in a uniform manner.

- **Symptoms:** Common symptoms include abdominal pain, bloody diarrhea, rectal bleeding, urgency to have bowel movements, and a feeling of incomplete evacuation.

- **Complications:** Severe cases might lead to colon perforation, increased risk of colon cancer, and extraintestinal complications like joint pain or skin lesions.

Crohn's Disease:

- **Location of Inflammation:** Can affect any part of the digestive tract from mouth to anus, often involving patches of inflamed tissue with healthy tissue in between.

- **Nature of Inflammation:** Inflammation can penetrate the entire thickness of the bowel wall, leading to deeper ulcers.

- **Symptoms:** Include abdominal pain, diarrhea, weight loss, fatigue, fever, and in some cases, can cause complications such as strictures, fistulas, or abscesses.

- **Complications:** May lead to bowel obstructions, malnutrition, fistulas, and complications beyond the digestive tract, such as arthritis or eye inflammation.

2.2 Symptoms and Triggers of Colitis

Symptoms:

- **Gastrointestinal Symptoms:** Abdominal pain or cramping, diarrhea, rectal bleeding, urgency to have bowel movements, and the sensation of incomplete evacuation.

- **Systemic Symptoms:** Fatigue, weight loss, fever, and decreased appetite can accompany severe flare-ups.

- **Extraintestinal Symptoms:** Joint pain, skin problems, and eye inflammation might occur in some cascs.

Triggers:

- **Dietary Triggers:** Certain foods may trigger or exacerbate colitis symptoms. These can vary widely among individuals and commonly include high-fiber foods, spicy dishes, dairy products, caffeine, alcohol, and fatty foods.

- **Stress:** Emotional stress or high-stress situations can contribute to flare-ups or worsen symptoms in some individuals.

- **Medication or Infections:** Changes in medications or exposure to infections might lead to increased inflammation and trigger colitis flare-ups.

2.3 Impact of Diet on Colitis Flare-Ups

Dietary Factors:

- **Trigger Foods:** Certain foods, as mentioned earlier, can exacerbate colitis symptoms by triggering inflammation in the gut or causing irritation.

- **Anti-Inflammatory Foods:** Conversely, some foods possess anti-inflammatory properties and may help reduce inflammation in the gut, potentially mitigating the frequency or severity of flare-ups.

- **Individual Variability:** The impact of diet on flare-ups varies from person to person due to individual sensitivities and tolerances. Identifying trigger foods and adopting a personalized diet is crucial in managing and preventing flare-ups.

Diet Modification for Flare-Up Management:

- During flare-ups, individuals often opt for a low-residue diet, which limits high-fiber foods to reduce bowel stimulation and irritation.

- Adjusting the diet to include easily digestible foods, avoiding known trigger foods, and opting for smaller, frequent meals might help manage symptoms during flare-ups.

Understanding the distinctions between ulcerative colitis and Crohn's disease, recognizing their symptoms and triggers, and comprehending the impact of diet on flare-ups are essential components in managing colitis effectively. Tailoring diet modifications based on individual needs and responses forms a crucial aspect of managing and mitigating flare-ups in individuals with colitis.

CHAPTER 3

Recommended Foods for Colitis

3.1 Easily Digestible Foods for Colitis

During periods of flare-ups or when experiencing digestive discomfort, incorporating easily digestible foods can help alleviate symptoms and reduce irritation in the gastrointestinal tract. Here are some recommended options:

1. White Rice:

- Easily digestible and gentle on the stomach.

- Provides carbohydrates for energy without overstimulating the digestive system.

2. Cooked Potatoes:

- Boiled or mashed potatoes are easy to digest.

- They offer a good source of potassium and vitamins.

3. Well-Cooked Vegetables:

- Carrots, zucchini, spinach, and green beans when thoroughly cooked can be easier on the digestive system.

- Avoid raw or fibrous vegetables during flare-ups.

4. Ripe Bananas:

- High in potassium and soluble fiber, which can help ease bowel movements.

- Provide a natural source of energy without causing irritation.

5. Applesauce:

- Contains soluble fiber and can be soothing to the digestive tract.

- Opt for peeled, cooked apples or unsweetened applesauce.

6. Lean Protein Sources:

- Skinless poultry, fish, or eggs can provide protein without being too taxing on digestion.

- Ensure they are cooked thoroughly and consumed in moderation.

7. Oatmeal:

- Cooked oats are gentle on the stomach and provide soluble fiber.

- Avoid adding high-fiber toppings during flare-ups.

8. Low-Lactose Dairy or Alternatives:

- Lactose-free milk, yogurt, or lactose-free dairy substitutes can be easier to digest for some individuals.

- Experiment to find suitable options that do not exacerbate symptoms.

9. White Bread or Crackers:

- Opt for refined grain products when dealing with digestive distress.

- These items are generally easier to digest compared to whole grain products.

10. Nut Butters:

- Smooth nut butters (without added sugars or seeds) can offer protein and healthy fats without being too harsh on the digestive system.

General Tips:

- **Cooking Methods:** Opt for steaming, boiling, or baking instead of frying or grilling to make foods easier to digest.

- **Small and Frequent Meals:** Eating smaller, more frequent meals throughout the day can ease the digestive load.

- **Hydration:** Stay adequately hydrated with water or herbal teas to support digestion.

These easily digestible food options can provide nourishment while minimizing irritation to the digestive tract during periods of colitis flare-ups or when experiencing gastrointestinal discomfort. However, individual tolerances may vary, so it's essential to identify specific triggers and preferences through personal experimentation and monitoring.

3.2 Nutrient-Dense Options

When managing colitis, incorporating nutrient-dense foods is crucial to maintain overall health and support the body's nutritional needs. Here are some nutrient-dense options beneficial for individuals with colitis:

Nutrient-Dense Options for Colitis:

1. Salmon and Other Fatty Fish:

- Rich in omega-3 fatty acids, which possess anti-inflammatory properties.

- Provides high-quality protein and essential nutrients like vitamin D.

2. Cooked Leafy Greens:

- Spinach, kale, and Swiss chard are packed with vitamins A, C, and K.

- Boil or steam them well to enhance digestibility.

3. Colorful Berries:

- Blueberries, raspberries, and strawberries offer antioxidants and vitamins.

- Can be blended into smoothies or eaten as a snack.

4. Sweet Potatoes:

- High in vitamins A and C, potassium, and fiber.

- Baking or boiling them makes them easier to digest.

5. Lean Protein Sources:

- Skinless poultry, lean cuts of beef, or tofu provide protein without excess fat.

- Choose grilled, baked, or boiled options.

6. Quinoa:

- A complete protein source with essential amino acids.

- Easier to digest compared to some other grains.

7. Greek Yogurt (if tolerated):

- High in protein, calcium, and probiotics.

- Opt for low-fat or lactose-free options if dairy is well-tolerated.

8. Eggs:

- A good source of protein, vitamins, and minerals.

- Easily digestible and versatile for different meal options.

9. Avocado:

- Provides healthy fats, fiber, potassium, and vitamins.

- Can be mashed and added to various dishes.

10. Almond Butter or Almonds:

- Offers healthy fats, protein, and vitamin E.

- Choose smooth almond butter without added sugars or salt.

Guidelines for Nutrient-Dense Foods:

- **Moderation:** While nutrient-dense foods are beneficial, moderation is key, especially during flare-ups. Monitor how your body responds to different foods.

- **Diversity:** Aim for a diverse range of nutrient-dense foods to ensure you get a variety of vitamins, minerals, and antioxidants.

- **Preparation Methods:** Opt for easily digestible preparations like steaming, baking, or blending to make these foods more gentle on the digestive system.

- **Hydration:** Adequate hydration is crucial to support digestion and nutrient absorption.

Incorporating these nutrient-dense options into your diet can help provide essential nutrients, support overall health, and aid in managing colitis. However, individual responses to these foods can vary, so it's essential to monitor how your body reacts to different nutrient-dense choices and adjust your diet accordingly. Consulting with a healthcare professional or a registered dietitian can also provide tailored guidance for your specific nutritional needs and colitis management.

3.3 Anti-Inflammatory Foods

Incorporating anti-inflammatory foods into your diet can potentially help manage colitis symptoms by reducing gut inflammation. Here are some anti-inflammatory options to consider:

Anti-Inflammatory Foods for Colitis:

1. Fatty Fish:

- Salmon, mackerel, sardines, and trout contain omega-3 fatty acids, known for their anti-inflammatory properties.

2. Berries:

- Blueberries, strawberries, raspberries, and blackberries are rich in antioxidants that combat inflammation.

3. Turmeric:

- Contains curcumin, a compound with potent anti-inflammatory effects. Use in cooking or consider supplements (consult a healthcare provider).

4. Ginger:

- Known for its anti-inflammatory and digestive properties. Use fresh or ground ginger in cooking or teas.

5. Leafy Greens:

- Spinach, kale, and Swiss chard contain vitamins, minerals, and phytochemicals that can reduce inflammation.

6. Extra Virgin Olive Oil:

- Rich in antioxidants and monounsaturated fats, it has anti-inflammatory effects. Use it for cooking or in dressings.

7. Nuts and Seeds:

- Walnuts, almonds, flaxseeds, and chia seeds provide omega-3 fatty acids and other anti-inflammatory compounds.

8. Tomatoes:

- High in lycopene, an antioxidant with anti-inflammatory properties. Enjoy them raw or cooked.

9. Green Tea:

- Contains catechins, which have anti-inflammatory effects. Drink as a soothing beverage.

10. Dark Chocolate (in moderation):

- High-quality dark chocolate with a high cocoa content contains flavonoids that possess anti-inflammatory properties.

Incorporating Anti-Inflammatory Foods:

- **Regular Consumption:** Aim to include these foods regularly in your meals to benefit from their anti-inflammatory properties.

- **Cooking Methods:** Prefer cooking methods that preserve nutrients and avoid excessive processing.

- **Balanced Diet:** Combine these anti-inflammatory foods with a variety of other nutritious options for overall health benefits.

While incorporating anti-inflammatory foods might help reduce inflammation and manage symptoms for some individuals, it's important to remember that responses can vary. Monitoring how your body reacts to these foods and consulting with a healthcare provider or a registered dietitian can provide personalized guidance in creating a diet plan that best suits your needs and supports colitis management.

3.4 Importance of Fiber in Colitis Diet

Fiber plays a crucial role in the diet, especially for individuals managing colitis.

However, its significance varies at different stages of the condition:

Importance of Fiber in Colitis Diet:

1. Balancing Gut Health:

- **During Remission:** Adequate fiber intake supports a healthy gut microbiome, promoting the growth of beneficial bacteria. This can help maintain intestinal health and prevent inflammation.

- **Source of Prebiotics:** Some types of fiber act as prebiotics, nourishing beneficial gut bacteria, which contribute to a balanced and thriving gut environment.

2. Regulation of Bowel Movements:

- **During Remission:** Fiber adds bulk to stools, aiding in regular bowel movements and preventing constipation. This can reduce the risk of complications like hemorrhoids or fissures.

- **Consideration during Flare-Ups:** In some cases, high-fiber foods can exacerbate symptoms during flare-ups. During these times, a low-residue or low-fiber diet might be recommended to minimize bowel irritation.

3. Impact on Inflammation:

- **Types of Fiber:** Soluble fiber, found in foods like oats, beans, and certain fruits, can help soothe and regulate the digestive system. It may reduce inflammation by forming a gel-like substance in the gut.

- **Insoluble Fiber:** While typically known for promoting bowel regularity, insoluble fiber in some cases can be more challenging to tolerate during flare-ups due to its potential to irritate the intestines.

4. Recommendations and Personalization:

- **Individual Response:** The tolerance to different types of fiber varies among individuals with colitis. Keeping a food diary to monitor how specific fiber-rich foods affect symptoms helps in personalizing the diet.

- **Gradual Introduction:** When reintroducing fiber after a flare-up, gradually incorporate it into the diet to assess tolerance levels and prevent discomfort.

5. Types of Fiber to Consider:

- **Soluble Fiber Sources:** Oats, psyllium husk, apples, oranges, berries, and certain vegetables like carrots and cooked spinach.

- **Insoluble Fiber Sources:** Whole grains, nuts, seeds, bran, and some vegetables like celery and raw leafy greens.

6. Professional Guidance:

- **Consultation with Healthcare Providers:** Seek guidance from healthcare professionals or a registered dietitian to determine the right balance of fiber in your diet. They can provide personalized recommendations based on your condition's severity and individual tolerances.

While fiber is generally beneficial for gut health, its role in colitis management requires a nuanced approach. Balancing the intake of soluble and insoluble fiber, monitoring personal responses, and seeking professional advice are key steps in leveraging the benefits of fiber while managing colitis effectively.

CHAPTER 4

Foods to Avoid with Colitis

4.1 Trigger Foods and Irritants

In managing colitis, identifying trigger foods and irritants can be crucial to reduce flare-ups and alleviate symptoms. Here are common foods that individuals with colitis might consider avoiding or limiting:

Foods to Avoid with Colitis:

1. High-Fiber Foods:

- **Raw Vegetables:** Raw vegetables, especially with tough skins or seeds, can be hard to digest and might aggravate the digestive system.

- **Whole Grains:** Whole grain products like whole wheat bread, brown rice, and high-fiber cereals can be challenging during flare-ups.

2. Dairy Products:

- **Lactose:** Some individuals with colitis might be lactose intolerant, leading to symptoms like gas, bloating, or diarrhea. Avoid or limit dairy if it triggers discomfort.

3. Spicy Foods:

- **Hot Peppers:** Spicy foods, particularly those containing hot peppers or strong spices, can irritate the digestive tract and lead to increased bowel movements or discomfort.

4. High-Fat Foods:

- **Fried Foods:** High-fat foods, especially fried items, can be harder to digest and might worsen symptoms or trigger flare-ups.

5. Caffeine and Alcohol:

- **Caffeinated Beverages:** Coffee, tea, and some sodas containing caffeine can stimulate the intestines, causing diarrhea or irritation.

- **Alcohol:** Alcoholic beverages can irritate the digestive tract and worsen symptoms for some individuals.

6. Carbonated Drinks:

- **Sodas and Sparkling Beverages:** Carbonated drinks might cause gas and bloating, leading to discomfort in the gastrointestinal tract.

7. High-Sugar Foods:

- **Refined Sugars:** Foods high in refined sugars, such as candies, pastries, and sugary cereals, might exacerbate symptoms for some individuals.

8. Artificial Sweeteners:

- **Sugar Alcohols:** Certain artificial sweeteners like sorbitol, commonly found in sugar-free gum and candies, can cause digestive upset in some people.

9. Seeds and Nuts:

- **Whole Seeds:** Seeds and nuts, especially when not thoroughly chewed, might irritate the digestive tract due to their rough texture.

10. Raw Fruits:

- **Some Raw Fruits:** Citrus fruits, apples with skin, and other raw fruits high in insoluble fiber might trigger discomfort during flare-ups.

Personalization and Observation:

- **Keep a Food Diary:** Monitor how specific foods affect your symptoms and consider eliminating or reducing those that consistently cause discomfort.

- **Gradual Reintroduction:** If eliminating certain foods, reintroduce them gradually to assess tolerance levels and potential triggers.

Understanding individual sensitivities and triggers is essential in managing colitis effectively. While these foods are commonly associated with triggering symptoms, individual responses can vary. It's important to work with healthcare providers or a registered dietitian to personalize dietary recommendations based on your specific condition and responses to food.

4.2 High-Fat and Spicy Foods

Avoiding high-fat and spicy foods can be beneficial for individuals managing colitis as these types of foods might exacerbate symptoms or trigger discomfort. Here are specific examples of high-fat and spicy foods to consider avoiding or limiting:

High-Fat Foods to Avoid with Colitis:

1. Fried Foods:

- **French Fries:** Deep-fried foods like fries contain high amounts of saturated fats that can be hard to digest and might worsen symptoms.

2. Fatty Meats:

- **Red Meat:** High-fat cuts of beef or pork can be harder on the digestive system. Opt for lean cuts if consumed.

- **Processed Meats:** Sausages, bacon, and deli meats often contain high levels of fat and might cause digestive issues.

3. Creamy or Rich Sauces:

- **Cream-Based Sauces:** Creamy pasta sauces, Alfredo, or creamy soups can be high in fat and might trigger discomfort.

4. Butter and Margarine:

- **Butter:** High-fat spreads or cooking fats like butter can be hard on the digestive tract.

- **Margarine:** Some margarines might contain trans fats, which can be detrimental to gut health.

5. Full-Fat Dairy Products:

- **Whole Milk:** Full-fat dairy products like whole milk, full-fat yogurt, or cheese might aggravate symptoms due to their high-fat content.

Spicy Foods to Avoid with Colitis:

1. Hot Peppers and Spicy Sauces:

- **Chili Peppers:** Hot peppers and spicy sauces can irritate the gastrointestinal tract and lead to discomfort or increased bowel movements.

2. Strong Spices:

- **Cayenne, Curry, or Paprika:** Strong spices used in various cuisines might cause irritation in the gut for some individuals.

3. Spicy Snacks:

- **Spicy Chips or Snacks:** Snacks coated with spicy seasonings can potentially aggravate symptoms.

4. Mexican or Thai Cuisine (varies):

- **Spicy Dishes:** Traditional dishes from cuisines like Mexican or Thai might contain spices or peppers that can trigger discomfort.

5. Buffalo Sauce and Hot Wings:

- **Hot Sauces:** Sauces like buffalo sauce used on wings or other dishes can be high in spice content and might cause gastrointestinal distress.

Observation and Customization:

- **Personal Responses:** Note how these foods affect your symptoms and consider eliminating or reducing those that consistently cause discomfort.

- **Customizing Diet:** Work with healthcare providers or a registered dietitian to tailor dietary recommendations based on your individual responses and the severity of your condition.

Avoiding high-fat and spicy foods can be a strategy to manage symptoms for some individuals with colitis. However, individual responses to these foods can vary, so it's essential to personalize dietary changes and seek guidance from healthcare professionals to create an effective and manageable diet plan.

4.3 Sugars and Artificial Sweeteners

Managing colitis often involves being mindful of sugars and artificial sweeteners, as they can potentially exacerbate symptoms for some individuals. Here are specific sugars and artificial sweeteners to consider limiting or avoiding:

Sugars to Avoid with Colitis:

1. Refined Sugars:

- **Candies and Sweets:** Confections high in refined sugars like candies, cookies, and pastries might trigger discomfort or worsen symptoms.

- **Sugary Beverages:** Soda, fruit juices, and energy drinks containing added sugars can cause gastrointestinal distress.

2. High-Fructose Corn Syrup (HFCS):

- **Processed Foods:** HFCS is commonly found in processed snacks, cereals, and sweetened beverages, which might exacerbate symptoms for some individuals.

3. Natural Sugars in Excess:

- **Excessive Fruits:** While fruits are nutritious, consuming excessive amounts, especially those high in natural sugars (e.g., mangoes, grapes), might cause digestive upset.

Artificial Sweeteners to Limit with Colitis:

1. Sorbitol and Mannitol:

- **Sugar-Free Gum and Candies:** These artificial sweeteners, found in some sugar-free products, can

cause gastrointestinal issues, such
as gas or diarrhea.

2. Aspartame:

- **Diet Beverages:** Aspartame,
  commonly found in diet sodas or
  sugar-free drinks, might cause
  discomfort in some individuals.

3. Saccharin:

- **Some Low-Calorie Foods:**
  Saccharin, found in some low-
  calorie or sugar-free products,
  might lead to gastrointestinal
  disturbances for certain individuals.

**Guidelines for Sugar and Sweetener
Consumption:**

- **Reading Labels:** Check food
  labels for hidden sugars or artificial
  sweeteners, especially in processed
  or packaged foods.

- **Moderation and Observation:**
  Monitor your body's response to
  different sugars and sweeteners.

Some individuals may tolerate certain types better than others.

- **Opting for Natural Sources:** When craving sweetness, consider natural options like small portions of fresh fruits or moderate amounts of natural sweeteners like honey or maple syrup if well-tolerated.

Managing sugar intake and being cautious with artificial sweeteners can be part of a dietary strategy to reduce symptoms and maintain gut health in individuals with colitis. However, responses to sugars and sweeteners can vary, so it's crucial to personalize dietary choices and seek guidance from healthcare professionals for tailored recommendations based on individual responses and overall health goals.

CHAPTER 5

Creating a Colitis-Friendly Meal Plan

5.1 Meal Planning Strategies

Creating a colitis-friendly meal plan involves thoughtful consideration of foods that are gentle on the digestive system while providing essential nutrients. Here are strategies to help craft a suitable meal plan for managing colitis:

Meal Planning Strategies for Colitis:

1. Emphasize Easily Digestible Foods:

- Prioritize foods that are gentle on the stomach, such as well-cooked vegetables, lean proteins, and easily digestible grains like white rice or oatmeal.

2. Opt for Small, Frequent Meals:

- Instead of large meals, consider eating smaller portions throughout the day to reduce digestive strain and manage symptoms better.

3. Include Low-Fiber Options:

- During flare-ups, focus on low-fiber or low-residue foods like peeled fruits, cooked vegetables, and refined grains to minimize bowel irritation.

4. Incorporate Protein Sources:

- Choose lean proteins like skinless poultry, fish, eggs, or tofu to ensure an adequate intake of essential nutrients without excessive fat content.

5. Add Gut-Friendly Foods:

- Include foods that support gut health, such as probiotic-rich yogurt (if tolerated), easily digestible fruits like bananas, and cooked vegetables.

6. Plan Balanced Meals:

- Aim for balanced meals comprising a protein source, easily digestible carbohydrates, and a small portion of healthy fats to provide sustained energy and nutrients.

7. Consider Cooking Methods:

- Opt for gentle cooking methods like steaming, boiling, or baking instead of frying or grilling to make foods more digestible.

8. Keep a Food Diary:

- Track your meals and symptoms to identify triggers or patterns, allowing you to adjust your meal plan based on what works best for your body.

9. Hydration is Key:

- Stay well-hydrated by consuming water, herbal teas, or diluted fruit juices to support digestion and prevent dehydration, a common concern with colitis.

10. Gradually Reintroduce Foods:

- When transitioning from a low-residue diet to a more varied diet, introduce new foods gradually to gauge tolerance levels and minimize discomfort.

Consultation with Professionals:

- **Registered Dietitian Support:** Seek guidance from a registered dietitian experienced in managing gastrointestinal conditions for personalized meal planning advice.

- **Healthcare Provider Input:** Discuss any dietary changes or concerns with your healthcare provider to ensure your meal plan aligns with your treatment plan.

A colitis-friendly meal plan revolves around selecting easily digestible, nourishing foods while minimizing potential triggers. Personalization and monitoring individual responses are key aspects in developing an effective and manageable meal plan for colitis management.

5.2 Sample Meal Ideas and Recipes

Here are some sample meal ideas and simple recipes suitable for a colitis-friendly diet:

Sample Meal Ideas:

Breakfast:

- **Banana Oatmeal:** Cooked oats with sliced ripe bananas, a drizzle of honey or maple syrup, and a sprinkle of cinnamon.

- **Scrambled Eggs:** Softly scrambled eggs with well-cooked spinach or mashed avocado on white toast.

Snacks:

- **Greek Yogurt Parfait:** Low-fat Greek yogurt with a handful of ripe berries and a sprinkle of granola (low in fiber).

- **Rice Cakes with Almond Butter:** Plain rice cakes spread with smooth almond butter.

Lunch:

- **Chicken and Rice Soup:** Clear chicken broth with shredded cooked chicken, white rice, and well-cooked carrots.

- **Tuna Salad:** Canned tuna with mashed avocado, served on white bread or crackers.

Snacks:

- **Applesauce:** Unsweetened applesauce or cooked, peeled apples.

- **Smoothie:** Blend ripe bananas, low-fat yogurt, and a splash of lactose-free milk or almond milk.

Dinner:

- **Baked Salmon:** Oven-baked salmon fillet with mashed sweet potatoes and steamed green beans.

- **Turkey and Mashed Potatoes:** Lean turkey cutlets with mashed potatoes made with low-fat milk or lactose-free options.

Simple Recipe: Chicken and Rice Soup

Ingredients:

- 2 cups cooked shredded chicken

- 4 cups low-sodium chicken broth

- 1 cup cooked white rice

- 1 cup diced carrots (cooked until soft)

- Salt and pepper to taste

- Fresh parsley (optional garnish)

Instructions:

1. In a pot, bring the chicken broth to a simmer.

2. Add the shredded chicken, cooked rice, and diced carrots to the broth.

3. Simmer for 10-15 minutes until flavors blend.

4. Season with salt and pepper to taste.

5. Garnish with fresh parsley if desired before serving.

Simple Recipe: Banana Oatmeal

Ingredients:

- 1 cup rolled oats

- 2 cups water or lactose-free milk

- 2 ripe bananas, sliced

- 2 tablespoons honey or maple syrup (optional)

- 1 teaspoon cinnamon (optional)

Instructions:

1. In a saucepan, bring water or milk to a boil.

2. Add the rolled oats and reduce heat to a simmer, stirring occasionally for 5-7 minutes.

3. Stir in sliced bananas and continue cooking until desired consistency.

4. Sweeten with honey or maple syrup, if desired, and sprinkle with cinnamon before serving.

These sample meal ideas and simple recipes prioritize easily digestible and low-irritant foods, suitable for managing colitis symptoms. Feel free to adjust ingredients based on personal tolerances and preferences, and always consult with a healthcare professional or a registered dietitian for personalized dietary recommendations.

5.3 Tips for Eating Out and Traveling with Colitis

Eating out and traveling with colitis requires some preparation and mindfulness to manage symptoms effectively. Here are tips to navigate dining out and traveling while managing colitis:

Tips for Eating Out:

1. Research Restaurants in Advance:

- Look for restaurants that offer easily customizable or bland options, such as grilled chicken or fish, white rice, steamed vegetables, or simple soups.

2. Communicate Dietary Needs:

- Inform restaurant staff about your dietary restrictions or preferences due to colitis. Request modifications like avoiding certain spices, sauces, or high-fiber ingredients.

3. Choose Simple Preparations:

- Opt for simple dishes that are easier on the digestive system, such as grilled or baked options rather than fried or heavily spiced meals.

4. Portion Control:

- Consider ordering smaller portions or appetizers to manage food intake and prevent overeating, which can trigger discomfort.

5. Pack Necessary Supplies:

- Carry digestive aids or medications prescribed by your doctor in case of unexpected flare-ups while dining out.

Tips for Traveling:

1. Plan Meals Ahead:

- Pack easily digestible snacks and meals for travel, such as rice cakes, bananas, low-fiber granola bars, or homemade sandwiches with lean protein.

2. Hydration is Key:

- Stay hydrated during travel by carrying a refillable water bottle and avoiding excessive caffeine or alcohol intake, which can dehydrate the body.

3. Research Local Cuisine:

- Learn about local cuisines and ingredients in your travel destination to make informed choices and identify potentially suitable dining options.

4. Pack a Travel Kit:

- Carry essentials such as wet wipes, hand sanitizer, extra medication, and a list of emergency contacts in case of unexpected flare-ups.

5. Plan Rest Stops:

- Plan rest stops during long journeys to manage restroom breaks and reduce stress, which can impact colitis symptoms.

General Tips:

1. Keep a Food Diary:

- Continue tracking your meals and any reactions to foods even while dining out or traveling to identify triggers and manage symptoms effectively.

2. Prioritize Rest and Relaxation:

- Maintain a balance between activities and relaxation to manage stress levels, which can affect colitis symptoms.

3. Consider Travel Insurance:

- When traveling long distances, consider travel insurance that covers unexpected medical situations, including exacerbations of colitis.

4. Seek Medical Advice:

- Before traveling, consult your healthcare provider for specific advice, necessary prescriptions, and recommendations tailored to your travel plans and health condition.

By planning ahead, communicating dietary needs, and staying mindful of triggers, you can better manage colitis symptoms while eating out or traveling. Flexibility, preparation, and maintaining open communication with restaurant staff or travel companions are essential for a smoother dining and travel experience.

CHAPTER 6

Lifestyle Modifications for Colitis Management

6.1 Stress Management Techniques

Managing stress is crucial in colitis management as it can impact symptom severity and frequency. Here are stress management techniques that can help individuals with colitis:

Stress Management Techniques:

1. Mindfulness Meditation:

- **Deep Breathing:** Practice deep breathing exercises to calm the nervous system and reduce stress.

- **Mindfulness Meditation:** Engage in guided meditation or mindfulness practices to stay present and alleviate anxiety.

2. Regular Exercise:

- **Low-Impact Activities:** Engage in low-impact exercises like yoga, walking, or swimming to release endorphins and reduce stress levels.

- **Strength Training:** Incorporate strength training or resistance exercises to boost overall well-being.

3. Relaxation Techniques:

- **Progressive Muscle Relaxation:** Practice tensing and relaxing different muscle groups to release tension.

- **Yoga and Stretching:** Gentle stretching and yoga poses can promote relaxation and reduce stress.

4. Time Management:

- **Prioritize Tasks:** Organize tasks and responsibilities to manage stress associated with overwhelming schedules.

- **Time for Rest:** Ensure sufficient time for rest and relaxation between tasks or activities.

5. Social Support:

- **Support Groups:** Join colitis support groups or communities to connect with others facing similar challenges.

- **Talk to Loved Ones:** Communicate with friends, family, or a therapist to share concerns and receive support.

6. Relaxation Activities:

- **Engage in Hobbies:** Pursue activities like painting, gardening, reading, or listening to music to unwind and reduce stress.

- **Nature Walks:** Spend time outdoors in nature, which can have a calming effect on the mind.

7. Healthy Lifestyle Choices:

- **Balanced Diet:** Maintain a nutritious diet as certain foods can impact stress levels and gut health.

- **Adequate Sleep:** Prioritize quality sleep to support overall well-being and reduce stress.

8. Mind-Body Practices:

- **Biofeedback:** Explore biofeedback techniques to gain awareness and control over bodily responses to stress.

- **Acupuncture or Massage:** Consider alternative therapies like acupuncture or massage for stress relief.

Integrating Stress Management:

- **Consistency:** Incorporate these techniques regularly into your routine for long-term stress management.

- **Personalization:** Experiment with different methods to find what works best for you.

- **Seek Professional Help:** Consider therapy or counseling to develop coping strategies tailored to your specific stress triggers and lifestyle.

Stress management isn't just about relaxation; it's about finding techniques that suit your lifestyle and effectively reduce stress. By incorporating these strategies, individuals with colitis can better manage stress, potentially reducing the frequency and severity of flare-ups.

6.2 Importance of Hydration

Hydration is paramount for individuals managing colitis as it supports overall health and aids in managing symptoms. Here's why adequate hydration is crucial in colitis management:

Importance of Hydration in Colitis:

1. Fluid Balance:

- **Maintains Fluid Levels:** Proper hydration helps maintain the body's fluid balance, crucial for overall bodily functions and digestion.

2. Bowel Function:

- **Prevents Dehydration:** Adequate hydration prevents dehydration, which can worsen symptoms like constipation or diarrhea commonly associated with colitis.

- **Softens Stool:** Proper hydration softens stool consistency, aiding in easier bowel movements and reducing discomfort.

3. Replenishes Losses:

- **During Flare-Ups:** Episodes of diarrhea or increased bowel movements lead to fluid loss. Adequate hydration helps replenish lost fluids and prevents dehydration.

4. Supports Healing:

- **Promotes Healing:** Hydration supports the healing process in the gastrointestinal tract, potentially reducing irritation and inflammation.

5. Improves Medication Effectiveness:

- **Enhances Medication Absorption:** Proper hydration can enhance the absorption of medications prescribed for colitis management.

6. Overall Health Benefits:

- **Boosts Energy Levels:** Being well-hydrated can help maintain energy levels and combat fatigue often associated with colitis and its symptoms.

- **Supports Immune Function:** Proper hydration supports immune function, aiding in the body's defense against infections or complications.

Hydration Tips for Colitis Management:

1. Drink Plenty of Fluids:

- **Water:** Aim for at least 8-10 cups of water daily, adjusting intake based on individual needs and activity levels.

- **Herbal Teas:** Opt for caffeine-free herbal teas or diluted fruit juices for variety and added hydration.

2. Monitor Urine Color:

- **Check Hydration Levels:** Monitor urine color; pale yellow indicates adequate hydration, while darker urine may signify dehydration.

3. Electrolyte Balance:

- **Include Electrolytes:** If experiencing diarrhea, consider replenishing electrolytes lost through sports drinks or oral rehydration solutions.

4. Spread Intake Throughout the Day:

- **Consistent Hydration:** Sip fluids steadily throughout the day rather than consuming large amounts at once to maintain consistent hydration levels.

5. Be Mindful of Triggers:

- **Avoid Irritants:** Choose non-irritating fluids; avoid highly caffeinated or sugary beverages that might exacerbate symptoms.

6. During Exercise or Hot Weather:

- **Increase Fluid Intake:** Drink extra fluids during physical activity or hot weather to compensate for increased fluid loss through sweating.

Adequate hydration is foundational for managing colitis symptoms and supporting overall health. Regularly drinking fluids can significantly impact digestive comfort, bowel regularity, and energy levels. Balancing hydration alongside dietary adjustments and other lifestyle modifications is essential for effective colitis management.

6.3 Incorporating Exercise into Daily Routine

Incorporating regular exercise into daily routines can be highly beneficial for individuals managing colitis. Here's why exercise is important and how to integrate it into your lifestyle:

Importance of Exercise in Colitis Management:

1. Stress Reduction:

- **Stress Relief:** Exercise can reduce stress levels, which is beneficial as stress can exacerbate colitis symptoms.

2. Improved Digestion:

- **Enhanced Bowel Function:** Regular physical activity can help regulate bowel movements and improve digestion.

3. Enhanced Well-Being:

- **Boosted Mood:** Exercise releases endorphins, promoting a sense of well-being and potentially alleviating feelings of anxiety or depression associated with colitis.

4. Weight Management:

- **Weight Control:** Maintaining a healthy weight through exercise can reduce the severity of colitis symptoms and support overall health.

5. Increased Energy Levels:

- **Boosted Energy:** Regular exercise can increase energy levels, combating fatigue often experienced by individuals with colitis.

Tips for Incorporating Exercise:

1. Choose Suitable Activities:

- **Low-Impact Exercises:** Opt for low-impact activities like walking, swimming, yoga, or cycling, which are gentle on the body.

2. Start Gradually:

- **Begin Slowly:** Start with shorter sessions and gradually increase the duration or intensity as fitness levels improve.

3. Consistency is Key:

- **Regular Routine:** Aim for consistency by scheduling regular exercise sessions throughout the week.

4. Listen to Your Body:

- **Pay Attention to Signals:** Be mindful of your body's signals; if a particular exercise exacerbates symptoms, consider alternative activities.

5. Mix Different Activities:

- **Variety:** Incorporate a mix of activities to keep it interesting and prevent monotony.

6. Prioritize Rest:

- **Rest Days:** Allow for rest days between workout sessions to prevent overexertion and facilitate recovery.

7. Consult a Healthcare Professional:

- **Health Advice:** Before starting any new exercise regimen, consult your healthcare provider to ensure it aligns with your current health status.

Simple Exercises for Colitis Management:

1. Walking:

- **Brisk Walks:** Take short brisk walks in nature or around your neighborhood to improve circulation and promote relaxation.

2. Yoga or Stretching:

- **Gentle Yoga Poses:** Engage in gentle yoga poses or stretching routines to promote relaxation and flexibility.

3. Swimming:

- **Low-Impact Aquatic Exercise:** Swimming or water aerobics can be gentle on the joints while providing a full-body workout.

4. Cycling:

- **Stationary or Outdoor:** Cycling on a stationary bike or outdoors can be a low-impact cardiovascular exercise option.

Integrating Exercise:

- **Personalization:** Find exercises that suit your preferences and fitness level.

- **Consistency:** Establish a routine that accommodates regular exercise without overexertion.

- **Gradual Progression:** Gradually increase intensity or duration as your fitness improves.

Regular exercise can play a significant role in managing colitis by reducing stress, improving digestion, and enhancing overall well-being. By integrating gentle and consistent physical activity into your routine, you can positively impact colitis symptoms and improve your quality of life.

CHAPTER 7

Supplements and Probiotics for Colitis

7.1 Role of Supplements in Colitis Management

Supplements can play a supportive role in colitis management, aiding in overall health, symptom alleviation, and potential modulation of the inflammatory response. However, it's important to consult with a healthcare professional before starting any supplement regimen. Here are some supplements that might be considered:

Role of Supplements in Colitis Management:

1. Omega-3 Fatty Acids:

- **Purpose:** Omega-3s have anti-inflammatory properties and might help reduce inflammation associated with colitis.

- **Sources:** Fish oil supplements or flaxseed oil capsules.

2. Vitamin D:

- **Purpose:** Vitamin D deficiency has been linked to increased inflammation. Supplementing might support immune function.

- **Sources:** Vitamin D3 supplements.

3. Probiotics:

- **Purpose:** Probiotics contain beneficial bacteria that can support gut health by promoting a balanced microbiome.

- **Sources:** Various probiotic supplements; strains and dosages may vary, so it's important to choose carefully.

4. Calcium and Vitamin D:

- **Purpose:** To support bone health, especially if corticosteroids are part of the treatment regimen.

- **Sources:** Calcium and Vitamin D supplements or combined formulations.

5. Iron:

- **Purpose:** If colitis leads to blood loss or anemia, iron supplements might be necessary to address deficiencies.

- **Sources:** Iron supplements, preferably under healthcare professional guidance to prevent digestive irritation.

Considerations for Supplements:

1. Healthcare Provider Guidance:

- **Consultation:** Discuss supplements with your healthcare provider to determine if they're suitable for your condition and any potential interactions with medications.

2. Quality of Supplements:

- **Choose Reputable Brands:** Opt for supplements from trusted brands to ensure quality and purity.

3. Personalization:

- **Tailored Approach:** Supplements' effectiveness can vary among individuals, so personalized recommendations are crucial.

4. Monitoring and Dosage:

- **Monitor Responses:** Keep track of how supplements affect your symptoms and well-being.

- **Correct Dosage:** Adhere to recommended dosages; excessive intake of certain supplements can have adverse effects.

5. Combination Therapies:

- **Synergistic Effects:** Some supplements might work synergistically with medications or other lifestyle modifications. Discuss potential combinations with healthcare providers.

Lifestyle Modifications vs. Supplements:

- **Comprehensive Approach:** Supplements should complement a holistic approach that includes dietary modifications, stress management, medication adherence, and regular medical check-ups.

While supplements might offer potential benefits in colitis management, they should be viewed as a complementary approach alongside other treatment strategies. Always seek guidance from healthcare professionals to ensure safe and appropriate use, as individual needs and responses can vary.

7.2 Recommended Probiotics and their Benefits

Probiotics are beneficial bacteria that can support gut health, potentially aiding in the management of colitis symptoms. Here are some recommended probiotics and their potential benefits:

Recommended Probiotics for Colitis:

1. **Lactobacillus acidophilus:**

   - **Benefits:** Known for its ability to produce lactic acid, promoting an environment unfavorable for harmful bacteria. It might help alleviate symptoms and maintain gut health.

2. **Bifidobacterium infantis:**

   - **Benefits:** This strain is believed to aid in balancing gut bacteria and modulating the immune system, potentially reducing inflammation in the gut.

3. Lactobacillus plantarum:

- **Benefits:** Recognized for its resilience in the gut environment, it may help reinforce the gut lining and contribute to a balanced microbiome.

4. Saccharomyces boulardii:

- **Benefits:** A yeast-based probiotic that might help restore the balance of gut flora disrupted by antibiotics and reduce diarrhea associated with colitis.

Benefits of Probiotics in Colitis Management:

1. Restoration of Gut Microbiota:

- Probiotics can restore the balance of beneficial bacteria in the gut, potentially reducing inflammation and improving digestive health.

2. **Immune Modulation:**

- They might modulate the immune response in the gut, potentially reducing inflammation associated with colitis.

3. **Reduced Symptoms:**

- Probiotics could alleviate certain colitis symptoms like diarrhea, abdominal discomfort, and bloating.

7.3 Consultation with Healthcare Professionals

1. **Importance of Professional Guidance:**

- Consulting with healthcare providers, especially gastroenterologists or registered dietitians, is crucial to determine the most suitable probiotic strains and dosages.

2. **Personalization and Monitoring:**

- Individual responses to probiotics can vary. Monitoring symptoms and responses while incorporating probiotics is essential for personalized care.

3. **Potential Interactions:**

- Discuss potential interactions with medications or other supplements to avoid adverse effects or diminished effectiveness.

4. **Choosing Quality Products:**

- Healthcare professionals can recommend trusted probiotic brands with proper strains and formulations.

5. **Combined Approach:**

- Probiotics should complement other colitis management strategies, including medication adherence, dietary adjustments, and stress management.

While probiotics offer potential benefits for managing colitis, their effectiveness can vary among individuals. Seeking guidance from healthcare professionals ensures the selection of appropriate probiotic strains, dosages, and a comprehensive approach tailored to your specific condition. Collaborating with professionals allows for the most effective and personalized management of colitis symptoms.

CHAPTER 8

Monitoring and Adapting the Colitis Diet

Monitoring and adapting the colitis diet is a crucial aspect of managing inflammatory bowel diseases like colitis. This process involves a multifaceted approach that includes keeping a detailed food diary, recognizing and effectively managing flare-ups, and making necessary adjustments to the diet based on individual responses and evolving health conditions.

8.1 Keeping a Food Diary

Maintaining a meticulous food diary is an invaluable tool in understanding the intricate relationship between diet and colitis symptoms. Individuals with colitis should record every meal, snack, and beverage consumed, along with the timing of ingestion. Additionally, it's important to note any symptoms experienced, such as abdominal pain, changes in bowel habits, fatigue, or other relevant indicators of colitis activity.

The food diary serves several purposes. Firstly, it helps identify potential trigger foods or patterns that correlate with symptom exacerbation. By establishing a comprehensive record of dietary intake and symptoms, individuals, along with healthcare providers, can discern trends and make informed decisions about which foods may be contributing to flare-ups.

8.2 Recognizing and Managing Flare-Ups

Recognition of colitis flare-ups is pivotal in implementing timely interventions to mitigate symptoms and prevent further exacerbation of the condition. Symptoms of a flare-up can vary but may include increased frequency of bowel movements, urgency, rectal bleeding, abdominal cramping, and fatigue. Individuals should be attuned to their bodies, promptly noting changes in symptoms, and reporting them to their healthcare team.

Managing flare-ups involves a combination of dietary adjustments, potential medication modifications (under the guidance of a healthcare professional), and lifestyle modifications. The information gleaned from the food diary plays a crucial role in this process, enabling individuals to correlate specific dietary factors with flare-ups and facilitating more targeted interventions.

8.3 Adjusting the Diet as Needed

Adapting the colitis diet is not a one-size-fits-all endeavor. Based on insights gained from the food diary and the recognition of flare-ups, individuals may need to make personalized adjustments to their dietary plans. This could involve eliminating or reducing specific trigger foods, altering meal timings, or modifying the consistency and fiber content of the diet.

Consultation with a healthcare provider or a registered dietitian is paramount during this phase. These professionals can provide evidence-based guidance, ensuring that dietary modifications are both effective and nutritionally sound. Adjustments may be iterative, requiring ongoing monitoring and refinement to achieve an optimal balance between managing symptoms and maintaining nutritional adequacy.

The process of monitoring and adapting the colitis diet is a dynamic and collaborative effort between individuals and healthcare providers. Through keeping a food diary, recognizing flare-ups, and making informed adjustments, individuals can empower themselves in managing colitis effectively and enhancing their overall well-being. Regular communication with healthcare professionals ensures a holistic approach, integrating dietary modifications seamlessly into the broader framework of colitis management.

CHAPTER 9

Seeking Professional Guidance

Seeking professional guidance is paramount in the effective management of colitis, ensuring that individuals receive comprehensive care that addresses both the medical and dietary aspects of the condition.

9.1 Importance of Consulting a Healthcare Provider

Consulting a healthcare provider is the cornerstone of managing colitis. Gastroenterologists, internists, or other healthcare professionals with expertise in gastrointestinal disorders play a pivotal role in diagnosis, treatment, and ongoing monitoring of colitis. The importance of this professional relationship lies in the ability to tailor medical interventions based on the individual's specific condition, response to treatment, and overall health.

Healthcare providers can conduct thorough assessments, prescribe medications when necessary, and monitor the progression of the disease. They also help individuals navigate potential complications and provide guidance on when adjustments to medications or other interventions might be required. Regular check-ups allow for proactive management and early detection of any changes in the disease course.

9.2 Working with a Registered Dietitian

Collaboration with a registered dietitian is a complementary aspect of managing colitis, focusing on the crucial link between diet and symptom management.

Registered dietitians specialize in translating scientific nutrition information into practical, individualized dietary advice. Working with a dietitian provides several benefits:

- **Personalized Dietary Guidance:** Dietitians can assess an individual's nutritional needs, dietary preferences, and medical history to develop a customized and sustainable colitis-friendly eating plan.

- **Education and Empowerment:** Dietitians empower individuals by providing education on the role of nutrition in colitis management. This includes information on trigger foods, nutrient-dense options, and strategies for maintaining a balanced diet.

- **Continuous Support:** Regular consultations with a dietitian allow for ongoing support and adjustments to the dietary plan as

needed. This dynamic approach
ensures that the diet remains
tailored to the individual's evolving
health status and lifestyle.

9.3 Incorporating Medical Advice into Dietary Changes

Successful colitis management involves
the integration of medical advice into
dietary changes. It's crucial for individuals
to communicate openly with their
healthcare providers about their dietary
habits, challenges, and any perceived
correlations between food intake and
symptoms. This collaboration ensures that
dietary adjustments align with the overall
treatment plan and are implemented in a
safe and effective manner.

Incorporating medical advice into dietary
changes may involve:

- **Medication Considerations:**
  Understanding how dietary changes

interact with prescribed
medications and whether any
modifications are needed to ensure
optimal therapeutic outcomes.

- **Monitoring Progress:** Regular
communication with healthcare
providers allows for the monitoring
of progress, making it possible to
assess the impact of dietary
changes on symptoms and adjust
the treatment plan accordingly.

- **Holistic Approach:** Recognizing
that the management of colitis
requires a holistic approach,
combining medical interventions,
dietary modifications, and lifestyle
adjustments for comprehensive
care.

seeking professional guidance is a
cornerstone of effective colitis
management. Through collaboration with
healthcare providers and registered
dietitians, individuals can navigate the
complexities of the condition, receive

personalized care, and integrate medical advice seamlessly into their dietary changes. This collaborative approach empowers individuals to proactively manage colitis, enhance their quality of life, and work towards long-term well-being.

www.ingramcontent.com/pod-product-compliance
Lightning Source LLC
Chambersburg PA
CBHW060944260726
48661CB00005B/1748